NAILS

A Manual and Atlas
Kristian Thomsen

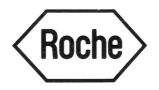

FADL Publishers
Prinsesse Charlottesgade 29
DK-2200 Copenhagen N
Denmark
FAX (+45) 35 36 62 29

Supported by an educational grant from
F. Hoffmann – La Roche Ltd, Basel, Switzerland

Preface

This manual and atlas of nail disorders is designed to provide dermatologists, general practitioners and medical students with clues to the diagnosis of the many nail changes they encounter when dealing with patients. It is my experience that many doctors, including dermatologists, are a little uncertain when they are confronted with nail problems, so I hope that this booklet will be of some help to them. It is based on many years of interest in nail disorders, this experience having given me something of a reputation as a nail specialist.

I wish to thank Dr Carsten Sand Petersen for encouraging me to write this book. Thanks are also due to F. Hoffmann-La Roche Ltd for its generous practical assistance.

Contents

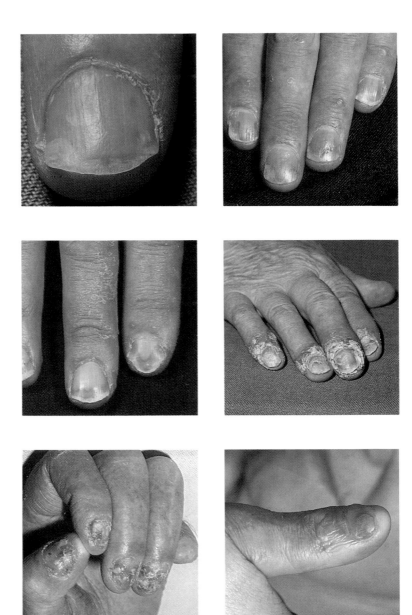

Psoriasis

The most characteristic feature of psoriasis of the nails is onycholysis with a yellow-brownish hue resembling that of apple jelly, the so-called oil spot (upper left). It is caused by the elevation of the nail plate by a psoriasis plaque in the nail bed. This feature is almost diagnostic. Pitting of the nail plate is frequent but is also seen in alopecia areata nails, onychomycosis, and eczema of the hand. It is caused by psoriatic involvement of the nail matrix (upper right, middle left).

Severe dystrophy caused by extensive involvement of the matrix is known as trachyonychia (middle right). The "nail splinters" that may be observed in these patients are subungual hemorrhages. Subungual pustules sometimes complicate pustular psoriasis and are also seen in acrodermatitis continua Hallopeau, where the final result is often severe atrophy of the nail and nail bed (bottom).

Treatment of nail psoriasis is difficult. Radiotherapy is useful in some cases, as is the injection of intralesional corticosteroid into the matrix. Nail changes may be so severe that systemic treatment is indicated, with either systemic retinoids or methotrexate. PUVA treatment is sometimes of benefit.

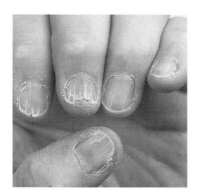 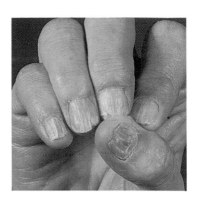

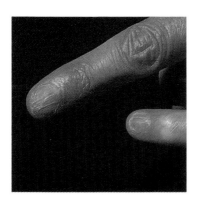

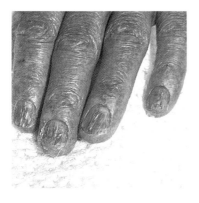

Lichen planus

In approximately 10% of patients with lichen planus, nails are involved, finger nails as well as toe nails. The nail plate is thinned with longitudinal ridges, and is therefore fragile. Sometimes koilonychia may even develop. In later stages of lichen planus there is a tendency to pterygium formation. In such cases the nail plate becomes divided into two parts by a scar-like formation growing from the proximal nail fold and inserting itself in the nail bed (middle). Lichen planus of the nails may ultimately lead to complete nail atrophy. These lesions of the nail are caused by involvement of the nail matrix. In some cases lichen planus is seated in the nail bed, resulting in a localized onycholysis, known as subungual lichen planus (bottom).

One, and sometimes the only way in which lichen planus manifests itself is twenty-nail dystrophy (see later). Nail changes identical to lichen planus are seen in graft-versus-host reaction following bone marrow transplantation and in systemic scleroderma, where they are indicative of an auto-immune reaction in the matrix.

Lichen planus nails are difficult to treat. Intralesional steroid injections into the nail matrix may be helpful as may radiotherapy. When systemic synthetic retinoids are used in the treatment of lichen planus, the nails are often improved.

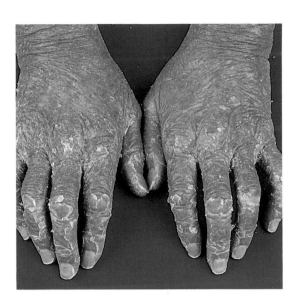

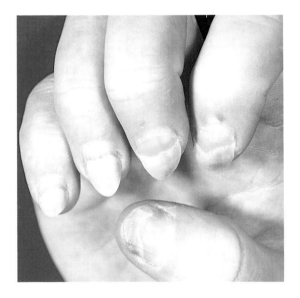

Pityriasis rubra pilaris

This rare, disabling skin disease, which is often of great thera-peutic concern, is always accompanied by nail alterations. The nails are thickened, and there is onycholysis with severe subungual hyperkeratosis and nail splinters. The nail sur-roundings are red and scaly.

These nail anomalies create great problems for the patients. The nails are difficult to cut and the handling of small objects, papers and the like is almost impossible.

Improvement occurs following treatment with synthetic retinoids, methotrexate or azathioprine.

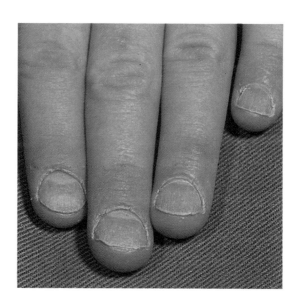

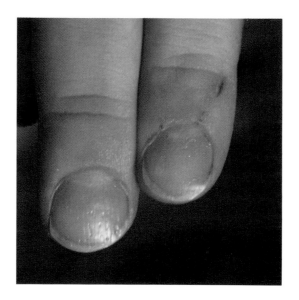

Alopecia areata

Nail changes are frequently seen in this apparently autoimmune condition, thus illustrating the fact that nails and hair are closely related structures. In a few cases, the nail changes have even preceded the alopecia.

Typically, a fine pitting of the nail plate is seen, sometimes arranged in a linear pattern. The lunula is often stippled, and red lunulae are an infrequent but striking sign.

If the hair regrows, the nails usually become normal again.

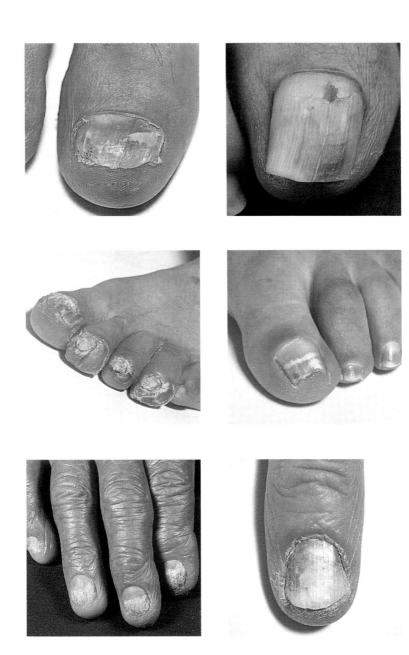

Fungal Infections

The big toe nail is usually the first nail to be infected, often preceded by an injury to the nail. However, all the toe nails can be infected and sometimes also many of the finger nails. Among the dermatophytes, *Trichophyton rubrum* is the commonest infecting organism while *Candida albicans* infection is often the cause of infection of the finger nails (bottom left). Usually the fungus first invades the nail bed and then spreads through the nail. In rare cases the infection is dorsal or superficial, giving rise to the clinical picture of leuconychia trichophytica (bottom right). The characteristic appearance of a fungus-infected nail is otherwise subungual hyperkeratosis with thickening and brownish discoloration of the nail plate, which becomes porous and easily breaks off. Sometimes it is difficult to distinguish between psoriasis of the nail and fungus infection but the characteristic demarcated onycholysis of psoriasis with a red-yellow halo, the so-called oil spot, is helpful. On the other hand, many psoriatic nails are often also the seat of a fungus infection.

Treatment of onychomycosis is systemic with griseofulvin or ketoconazol, though among older people the growth rate of the toe nails is so slow that treatment often proves ineffective. However, the new systemic antimycotics, terbinafine and itraconazole, penetrate the nail plate from the nail bed, so that the concentration of these drugs in the nail tissue is independent of the rate of nail growth.

Another new drug, amorolfine, a phenylpropyl morpholine, has been shown to be effective even in toe nail onychomycosis when used as a 5% nail lacquer.

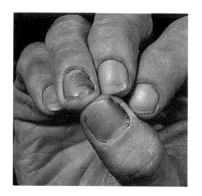
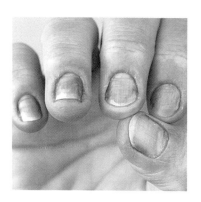
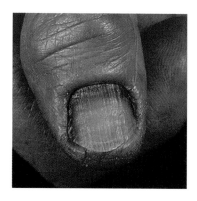

Chronic Paronychia

In chronic paronychia a mixed flora of microorganisms is found: *Candida albicans*, *Staphylococcus aureus* and *Pseudomonas*. There is chronic, red, tender swelling of the periungual tissue and the cuticula are absent, leaving an open passage to the compartment below the proximal nail fold. The matrix becomes involved and this causes characteristic transversal ridging of the nail plate, which is most pronounced at the lateral edges of the nail and is accompanied by a green-black discolouration due to *Pseudomonas*.

Chronic paronychia are mainly seen in young females whose work entails frequent wetting of the hands, e.g. nurses, cooks and florists. A predisposing factor is impaired peripheral circulation as in perniosis.

Treatment consists in the application of topical and systemic antibiotics, but avoiding excessive contact with water is of paramount importance.

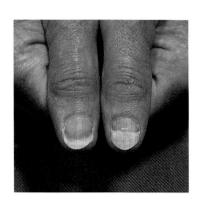 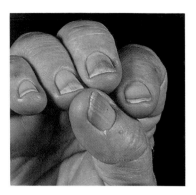

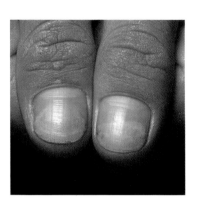 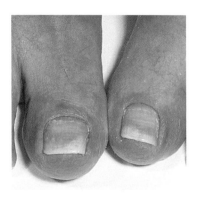

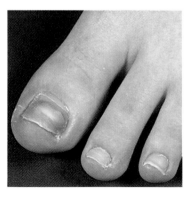

Onycholysis

Onycholysis is the separation of the nail plate from the nail bed. One or more nails may be affected and usually the condition is idiopathic. It can, however, be traumatic, for instance when the big toe nails are the site of distal onycholysis due to pressure from footwear (middle right, bottom). Prolonged immersion in water also may cause onycholysis.

Onycholysis is also seen in cases of hyperhidrosis, in thyreotoxicosis and accompanying other nail disorders such as psoriasis and fungus infection. Photoonycholysis occurs after the ingestion of phototoxic drugs such as dimethyl-chlortetracycline, and as a complication of PUVA therapy. In porphyria cutanea tarda and erythropoietic protoporphyria, photoonycholysis is a frequent phenomenon due to blister formation underneath the nail plate (upper right, middle left). This photoonycholysis is often very painful and can result in loss of the nail.

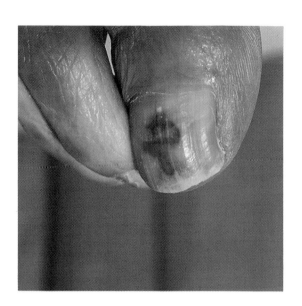

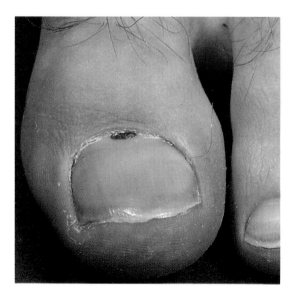

Hemorrhage

Splinters of the nail are small bleeding points between the ridges of the under side of the nail plate. As the nail grows, this hemorrhage is drawn distally by the moving nail, thereby forming a hemorrhagic line or "splinter". Splinters are most often of traumatic origin but they are also seen as a result of low oxygen tension following climbing in high mountains, and are present in many nail disorders such as psoriasis, chronic hand eczema, pityriasis rubra pilaris and onycho-mycosis.

In very rare cases, endocarditis lenta is the cause.

Subungual hematomas are also usually of traumatic origin but are sometimes a symptom of blood dyscrasias such as leukemia or bone marrow depression after chemotherapy. Subungual hematomas may mimic malignant melanoma due to the appearance of the "tricolore" sign.

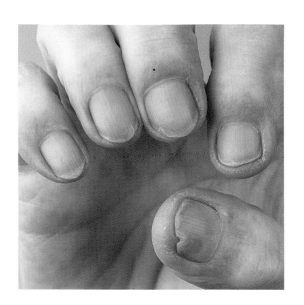

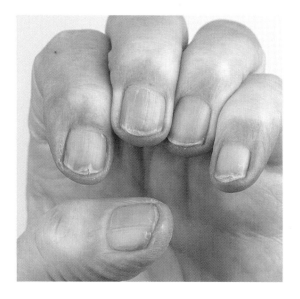

Brittle Nails

Brittle nails are extremely common, especially in women in their forties. It is caused by the frequent uptake of water and subsequent drying of the nail plate leading to changes of the keratin filaments in the nail. Most often a lamellar horizontal splitting of the distal edge occurs but isolated splits at the free edge are also sometimes encountered.

Certain types of varnish removers may aggravate this common condition. Treatment is difficult but consists in avoiding frequent contact with water and the use of emollients or vaseline. Over-enthusiastic manicure should also be avoided.

In rare cases iron deficiency is present and iron supplements may be beneficial. Administration of B vitamins or calcium is ineffective, but biotin seems to work.

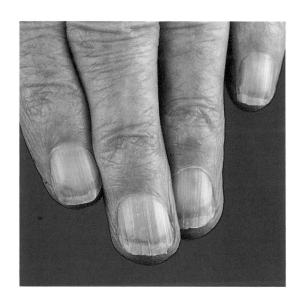

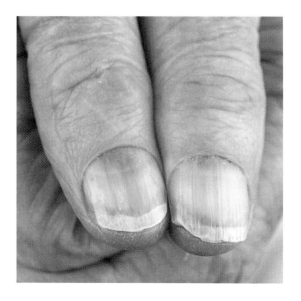

Nails in Old Age

Nail growth tends to decrease with age by up to one third from youth to old age. With age the nails become thin and brittle with a lustreless, grey surface and a darker distal band, the so-called Terry nails. "Half-and-half nails", in which the proximal part of the nail is grey and the distal part brown, are not uncommon in otherwise healthy elderly persons.

Normal nails have longitudinal ridges, but this phenomenon becomes more pronounced with age and the individual ridges often have a strikingly beaded appearance.

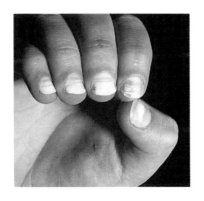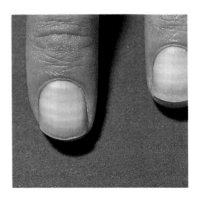

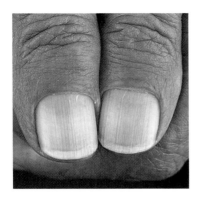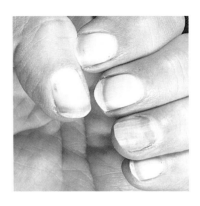

Leukonychia

Leukonychia, white nails, or white spots of the nails, is the most common discolouration of the nails. Often it is of traumatic origin due to disturbance of keratinization when the nail is formed, but congenital, autosomal dominant leukonychia exists with either diffuse whitening of the nail plate obscuring the lunula or with transverse white bands (upper left). The so-called Muercke's lines are also transverse, white lines but they are caused by hypoalbuminemia and are characteristically seen in patients with cirrhosis of the liver (upper right). Diffuse whitening of the nails is a frequent cutaneous marker of cirrhosis (bottom). Finally, transverse white bands corresponding to individual courses of chemotherapy are one of the more common side effects of systemic cancer chemotherapy, the number of white bands indicates the number of courses the patient has undergone. Systemic, synthetic retinoids may produce similar transverse, white banding.

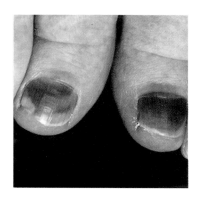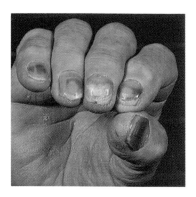
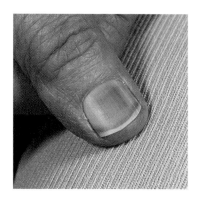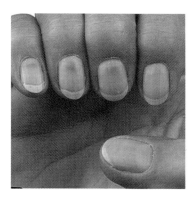

Black Nails

As mentioned previously, black discolouration of the nail can be caused by the pigment from *Pseudomonas* infection, but also by subungual hemorrhage following trauma (upper left). With the black "PUVA nails", the discolouration in the middle of the nail plate is also due to hemorrhage (bottom right).

Systemic chemotherapy can result in black or brown discolouration of the nails, particularly after bleomycin or adriamycin (upper right, bottom left). This colour change is caused by increased melanin formation in the matrix. An identical black pigmentation of the nail plate is occasionally seen in patients treated with acidothymidine. Radiotherapy of skin diseases of the fingers may result in a similar pigmentation.

Longitudinal black bands in the nail plate extending from the proximal nail fold to the distal edge of the nail are a frequent finding in black people. In white people, however, they are rare and indicate a naevocellular naevus or a malignant melanoma in the nail matrix. In such cases, therefore, biopsy should be performed.

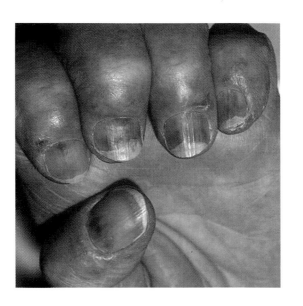

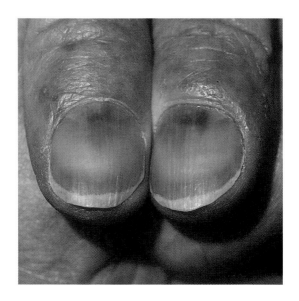

Red Nails

Red nails or red lunulae is a rare discolouration of the nail located in the proximal third of the nail plate with a blurred demarcation from the normally coloured distal part of the nail. The purplish colour is caused by hyperemia of the nail bed analogous to erythema palmare. It occurs in systemic lupus erythematosus, in alopecia areata and accompanying drug eruptions.

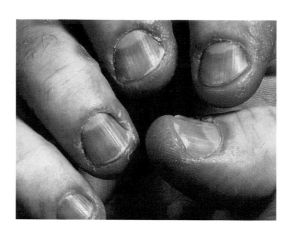

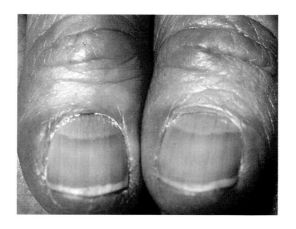

Blue Nails

"Azure blue lunulae" is another term for this nail manifestation of argyria. It may be seen in the absence of any other cutaneous signs of argyria. The colour is permanent but eventually deepens.

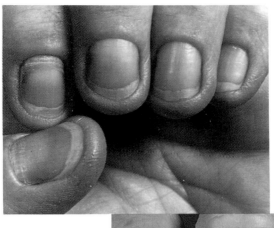

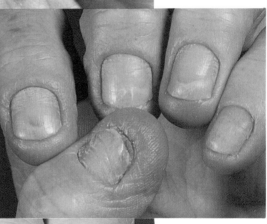

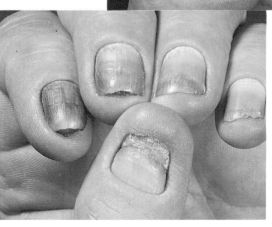

Yellow Nails

The striking sign of yellow nails appears when the nails stop growing. Patients with the yellow nail syndrome only have to cut their nails once or twice a year. In addition to the yellowish-green discolouration, the nail plate is thickened and the surface is smooth and curved in both axes. Cuticula are always absent. Finger nails as well as toe nails are affected.

Originally, lymphedema was thought to be the cause of this disease but often the cause is obscure. Pulmonary infections have been described in association with the syndrome and the last case we saw was a patient with pulmonary tuberculosis caused by *Mycobacterium avium*. Following antituberculous therapy, the patient's nails started to grow and finally became normal.

Unless an associated disease is successfully diagnosed and treated, treatment of idiopathic yellow nail syndrome is unrewarding.

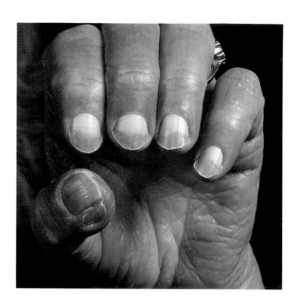

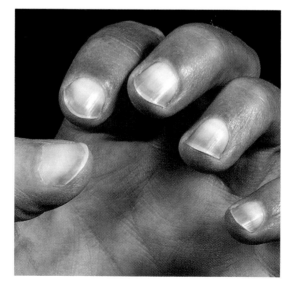

Half-and-Half Nails

In "half-and-half nails" the proximal part of the nail is white while the distal part is brown. This phenomenon is most often seen in patients with uremia but also following chemotherapy and sometimes as an age-related condition. Half-and-half nails have been observed in a few patients with AIDS.

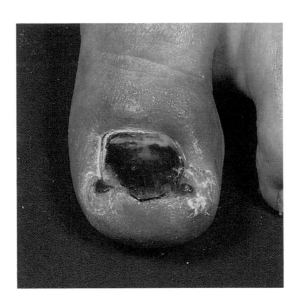

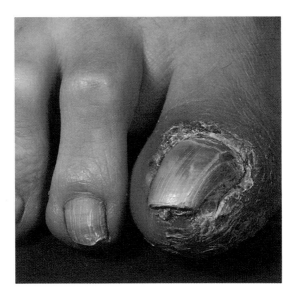

Ingrowing Toe Nails

Pressure from ill-fitting footwear is the cause of this painful inflammatory condition, which most often affects the great toe nails. Over-trimming of the lateral edges of the nails predisposes to ingrowing toe nails. Granulation tissue is formed at the lateral nail folds, causing a resemblance to pyogenic granuloma. If the adjacent nail is arched with overcurvature along the longitudinal axis, as is the case with pincer nails, the lateral edges of the nail plate easily penetrate the surrounding tissue and cause inflammation.

Conservative treatment consists of a change of footwear, correct nail cutting, the insertion of cotton wool under the free edge of the nail and the application of a nail brace to flatten the nail.

Surgical treatment consists of excision of the excess granulation tissue and, in recalcitrant cases, of lateral matrix resection to narrow the nail plate.

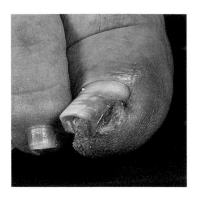 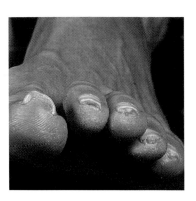

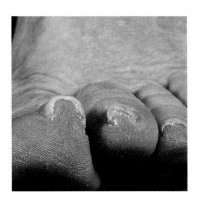 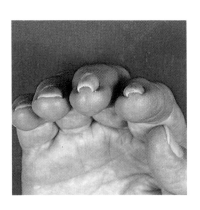

Pincer Nails

In pincer nails, also known as trumpet nails, there is a pronounced transverse overcurvature of the nails, especially on
the feet. In hereditary forms, the finger nails are also
involved. The lateral edges of the nail penetrate the
underlying soft tissue in a pincer-like fashion, causing
considerable pain. Pincer nails may be of traumatic origin due
to pressure from ill-fitting footwear, but are also seen in
psoriasis and following the use of some of the early beta-
blockers.

   Treatment, if indicated, consists of surgical resection of the
lateral parts of the nail matrix.

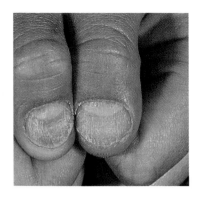 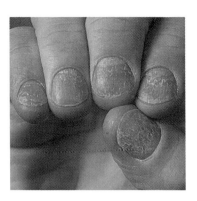

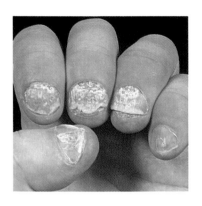 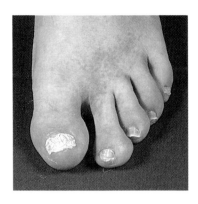

Twenty-Nail Dystrophy

This rather troublesome disease of all or almost all the finger and toe nails occurs mainly in children or adolescents. It is also referred to as excessive ridging of the nail plate, rough nails or trachyonychia. As these names imply, the nail surface is rough and ridged. The nail plate flattens and sometimes a few nails even present as koilonychia. The lunula is spotted or obscured. Histologic examination of matrix biopsies has shown lichen planus-like changes or spongiosis.

The etiology is unknown but sometimes twenty-nail dystrophy is seen in patients with lichen planus, psoriasis or alopecia areata. In a few cases we have even seen the nail changes precede areate alopecia.

Treatment is difficult but steroid injections into the matrix or superficial x-ray therapy may be helpful.

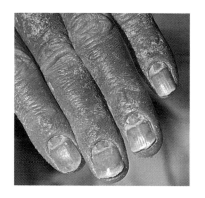 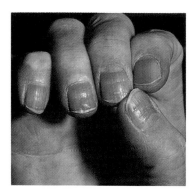

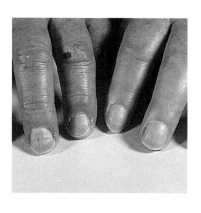 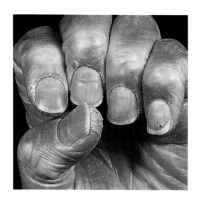

Beau's Lines

A few weeks after a severe illness, a transverse depression of the surface of all the nails appears at the basis of the nail, a sign named Beau's lines. This furrow moves distally as the nail grows. The furrow may be shallow or deep, sometimes even resulting in fracture of the nail plate.

This condition is caused by a maturity arrest of the nail forming cells in the matrix. It is seen after shock, coronary occlusion with hypotension, sepsis and severe skin diseases such as exfoliative erythroderma. Beau's lines may also be present in patients with severe zinc deficiency. Single or multiple Beau's lines regularly appear after cancer chemo-therapy.

Usually all the nails are affected but recently we saw a patient with erythroderma who also had a hemiparesis after a stroke. He developed Beau's lines only in the nails of the non-paralysed extremities.

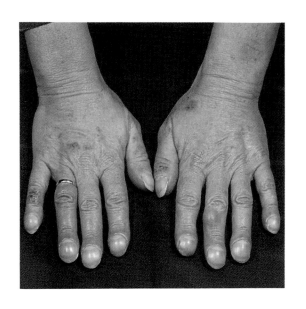

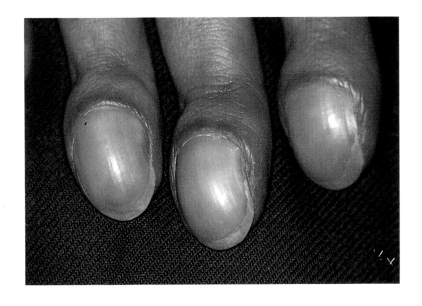

Clubbing

Finger nail clubbing, or hippocratic nails, is a well-known skin marker of internal disease. It accompanies chronic lung or heart disease with cor pulmonale, is seen in a more acute form in carcinoma of the lung, and is part of the thyreotropic syndrome together with malignant exophthalmus and pretibial myxedema. However, familial clubbing not associated with other diseases is quite common and it is worth asking whether family members have the same anomaly.

Clubbing is a major sign in hypertrophic pulmonary osteo-arthropathy.

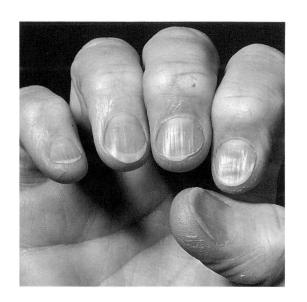

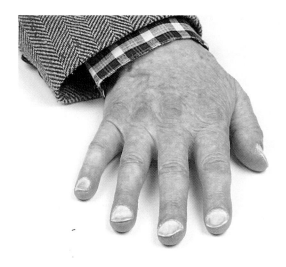

Spoon Nails

Also known as koilonychia, spoon nails are a condition in which the nail plate is very brittle, thin and flattened with slightly elevated edges. Finger nails as well as toe nails may be involved. It is a physiological phenomenon in the big toe nails of children below 2 years of age. A hereditary form of koilonychia is not uncommon, but several acquired forms also occur, namely in malnutrition, in thyreotoxicosis, in iron deficiency and as a feature of severe Raynaud's syndrome and scleroderma.

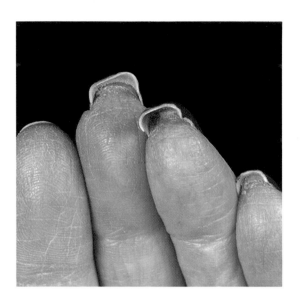

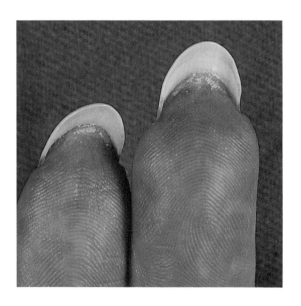

Pterygium inversum

Usually seen in systemic scleroderma, this anomaly of the nail is not uncommon in other conditions and is even seen in otherwise healthy persons. Pterygium inversum unguis, also known as ventral pterygium, is a fixation of the hyponychium (the distal part of the nail bed) to the underside of the distal part of the nail plate. In severe cases this results in an over-curvature of the nail. Owing to the tenderness of the abnormal hyponychial band, patients with this anomaly hesitate to trim their nails, preferring instead to wear long nails in order to protect the tender hyponychial tissue. As already mentioned, pterygium inversum is common in systemic scleroderma, but it is also seen in systemic lupus erythematosus, in dermatomyositis and in patients with Raynaud's phenomenon. However, healthy persons may exhibit this anomaly, often as a familial trait.

If the condition causes severe discomfort, excision of the abnormal hyponychial tissue may be considered.

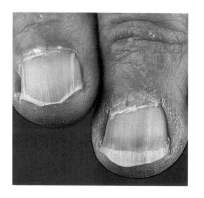 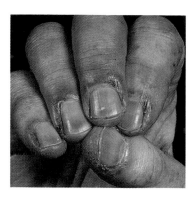

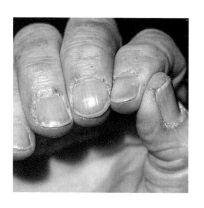 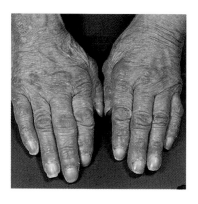

Nails in Dermatomyositis

Changes affecting the nails and their surroundings are almost obligatory when dermatomyositis is active. On the other hand, remission of the disease is accompanied by normalization of the very distinct nail picture. In dermatomyositis, the cuticula are widened and frayed at the edges and there is reddish cyanotic swelling of the proximal nail fold with telangiectasia and small thrombi. The dermal capillaries, which are horizontal in the proximal nail fold and which can be visualized by capillary microscopy, are greatly dilated and tortuous.

Pterygium inversum unguis is also a frequent finding in dermatomyositis.

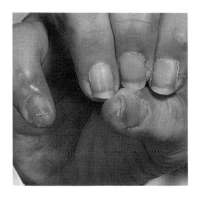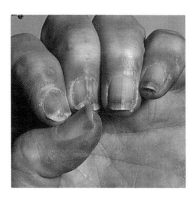
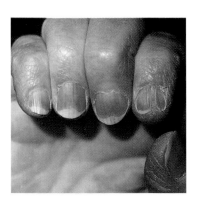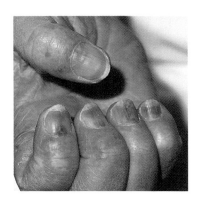

Nails in Systemic Lupus Erythematosus

The nail changes are similar to those encountered in dermato-myositis, with widening of the cuticula and swelling of the proximal nail fold with telangiectasia. In addition, however, vasculitis of the nail matrix causes severe nail dystrophy with deep longitudinal furrows which are sometimes permanent due to scarring of the matrix. Lupus erythematosus vasculitis in the nail bed gives rise to onycholysis.

Red lunulae are occasionally a sign of systemic lupus erythematosus, as is pterygium inversum.

Similar nail changes are also part of the clinical spectrum in mixed connective tissue disease.

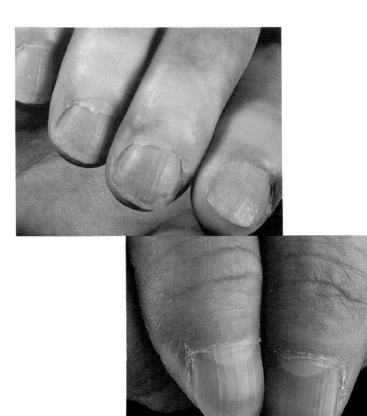

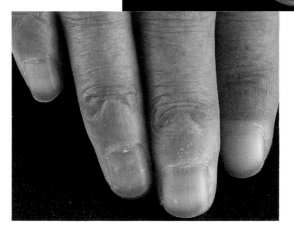

Nails in Scleroderma

Nail changes are common in systemic scleroderma with Raynaud's phenomenon. The nails diminish in size, and are thin and flat; sometimes spoon nails are seen. The finger nails may also, however, develop a claw-like appearance in scleroderma, with pronounced overcurvature of the nail plate along its longitudinal axis. Pterygium inversum unguis, a frequent phenomenon in this disease, gives rise to transverse overcurvature of the nail plate. Widening of the cuticula, which is a common nail change in dermatomyositis and systemic lupus erythematosus, is also seen in scleroderma.

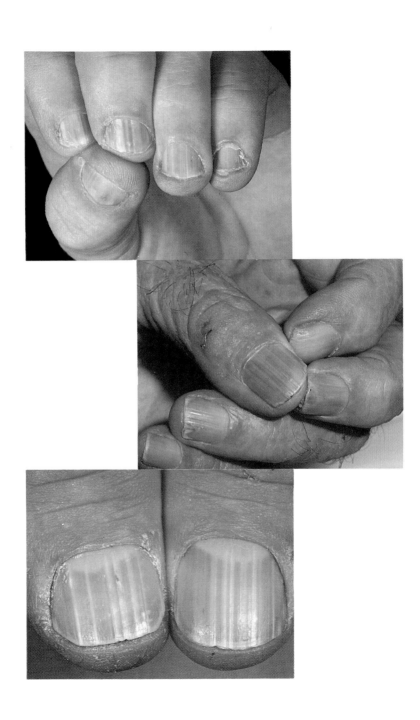

Nails in Darier's Disease

Almost all patients with dyskeratosis follicularis Darier
exhibit nail changes. There are single or multiple red or white
longitudinal streaks in the nail plate with distal subungual
keratosis, producing a small notch in the free edge of the nail
plate. These lines transverse the lunula right up to the
proximal nail fold. Identical nail changes are seen in patients
with benign familial pemphigus, Hailey-Hailey's disease. I
myself have observed this sign in 8 out of 9 patients with
Hailey-Hailey. The gravity of this nail sign does not parallel
the activity of the skin disease, and that holds for both
Darier's and Hailey-Hailey's diseases.

Retinoid treatment is effective against Darier's disease but
has no effect upon these nail changes.

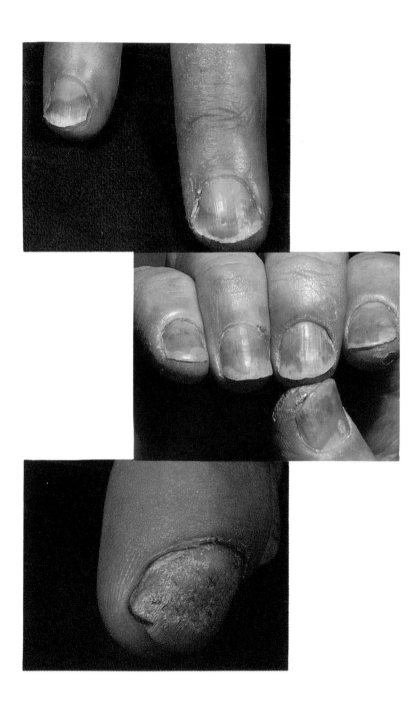

Nails in Reiter's Disease

The nail changes are similar to those seen in psoriasis. However, punched out deep pits in the nail plate, subungual pustules and periungual psoriasiform lesions are characteristic, diagnostic features. The affected nails are often extremely tender and painful.

Treatment with methotrexate may be indicated.

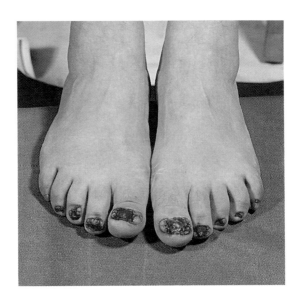

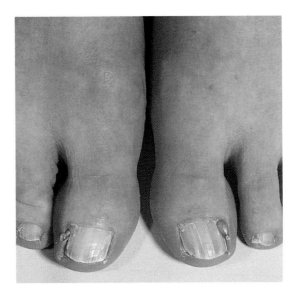

Nails in Tuberous Sclerosis

In tuberous sclerosis with mental deficiency, epilepsy and angiofibromas of the face, the characteristic nail changes are of diagnostic assistance. Wart-like periungual fibrous tumours known as Koenen tumours are found on the finger nails and, even more frequently, on the toe nails.

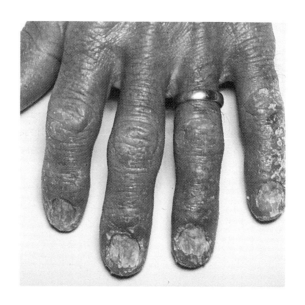

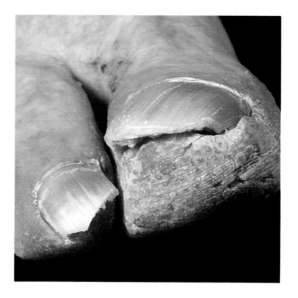

Nails in Basex Syndrome

Basex syndrome or acrokeratosis paraneoplastica is a paraneo-plastic syndrome with acral psoriasis-like lesions typically confined to the nose, cheeks, helices, fingers and toes associated with carcinomas of the rhinopharynx, esophagus or lungs. The nails demonstrate changes similar to those seen in matrix psoriasis with severe dystrophy and subungual hyperkeratosis.

Where the malignancy has been successfully treated, the skin and nail changes disappear only to recur again if the malignancy relapses.

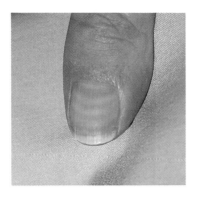

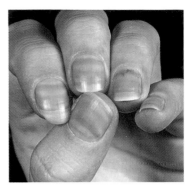

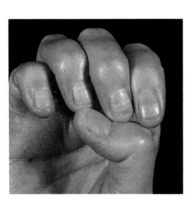

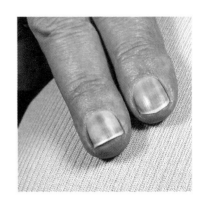

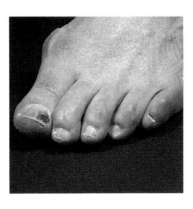

Chemotherapy Nails

One of the most common side effects of cancer chemotherapy is hair loss, both anagen and telogen. No less frequent but usually not recognized and less dramatic are nail changes. Multiple transverse white bands occur after cyclic chemotherapy, each band corresponding to a chemotherapeutic cycle (upper, middle left). Thus, simple inspection of the nail will reveal the number of cycles given. The white colouration is caused by defective keratinization due to cell arrest in the matrix. High-dose chemotherapy may produce Beau's lines, sometimes followed by nail loss.

Pigmentation of the nail plate, either diffuse or arranged in transverse or longitudinal bands, is caused by increased melanin formation by the matrix cells (middle right).

Pulse therapy with corticosteroids may produce dark banding as well. Acidothymidine used in the treatment of patients with AIDS has occasionally resulted in a similar melanonychia.

Subungual hemorrhage is common in patients undergoing chemotherapy, and is most often located on the big toe or the second toe due to trauma from the footwear. In such cases, subungual malignant melanoma is often a differential diagnosis (bottom).

We have encountered a few cases of acute paronychia after methotrexate, perhaps due to impaired immunity. Half-and-half nails, where the proximal part of the nail is white while the distal part is brown, are a not uncommon dermatological complication of cancer chemotherapy.

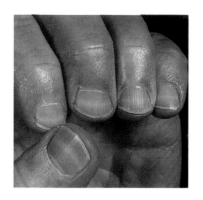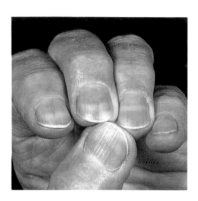
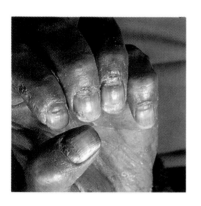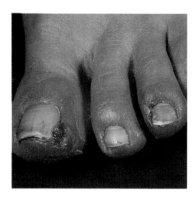

Retinoid Nails

Synthetic retinoids are now in widespread use in dermatology, isotretinoin in severe acne and rosacea, etretinate in psoriasis and various disorders of keratinization. Many cutaneous side effects are caused by these potent drugs, and hair and nails are also affected. The nails may become the site of transverse ridging, or transverse white banding (upper). Sometimes onychomadesis and even deep Beau's lines have been observed as a side effect of this novel group of drugs (bottom left). The most common side effect, however, is thinning of the nail plate with brittleness.

Acute paronychia, especially of the big toe, is a less frequent adverse reaction to the use of these retinoids, but is often very painful (bottom right). These nail changes will diminish or disappear when the dosage is reduced or the treatment discontinued.

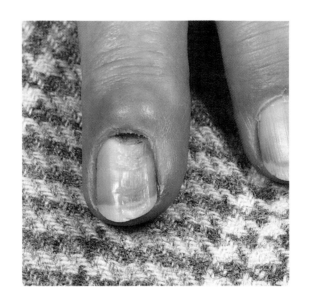

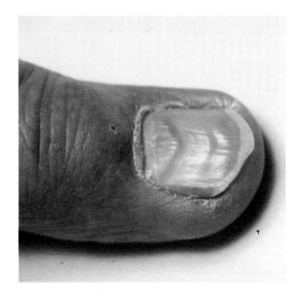

Mucoid Cysts

These small, firm, elastic cystic nodules are located on the proximal nail fold or on the dorsal aspect of the distal interphalangeal joint of one or several fingers. Due to pressure on the matrix, a longitudinal sulcus is formed in the nail plate; this may be the presenting sign of the tumour.

Therapy consists of puncture of the cyst with intralesional corticosteroid injection or excision.

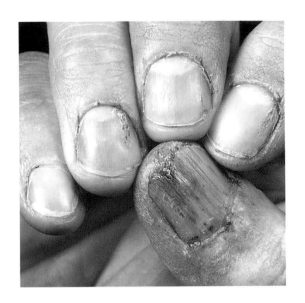

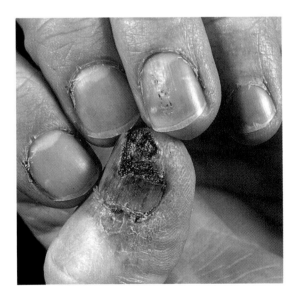

Subungual Warts

Not infrequently, benign or malignant tumours may be located underneath the nail plate in the nail bed. The most common of the benign subungual tumours is the viral wart, which may grow from its initial site in the periungual tissue into the nail bed, usually the distal part of the nail bed separating the nail plate from its bed.

Subungual warts are usually both painful and difficult to treat. In many cases, surgical treatment, with partial ablatio of the nail and curettage of the wart, is indicated.

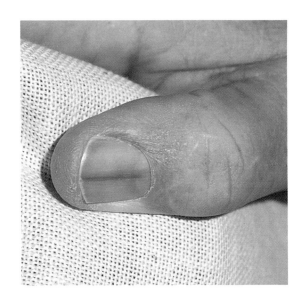

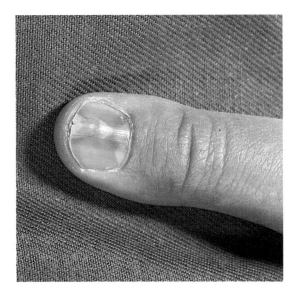

Subungual Fibromas

Subungual fibromas may form a longitudinal chord located on the underside of the nail and appearing at the distal edge of the nail plate as a small tuft, which grows with the nail. These fibromas originate in the matrix of the nail. Because of their dark colour, they may mimic melanocytic nevi.

Usually therapy is not indicated.

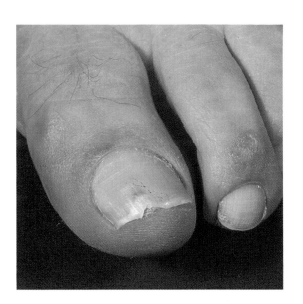

Subungual Exostoses

Subungual exostoses are osseous outgrowths from the distal phalanx forming a rounded, firm, subungual tumour which lifts the nail plate and sometimes destroys it. These painful tumours are rather common, especially in young people, and are usually located on the big toe. They can be visualized by x-ray examination. Therapy is surgical with excision of the exostosis.

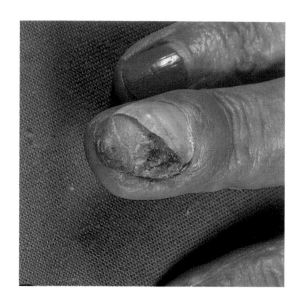

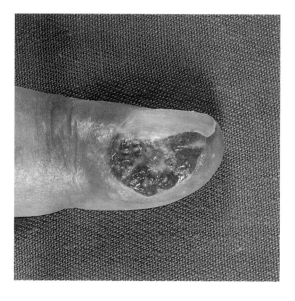

Subungual Squamous Cell Carcinoma

If this malignant tumour is located beneath the nail it is often misdiagnosed as a common wart, subungual exostosis or onychomycosis. It is a verrucous, scaly tumour which elevates and destroys the nail plate. It does not usually ulcerate and rarely metastasizes. Human papilloma virus is detected in squamous cell carcinomas of the finger nails with increasing frequency. Subungual squamous cell carcinoma may be preceded by subungual Bowen's disease, which is even more difficult to diagnose mainly because of a lack of signs and symptoms.

Treatment consists in excision or in amputation of the finger.

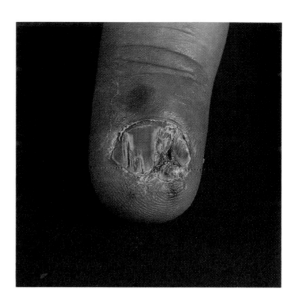

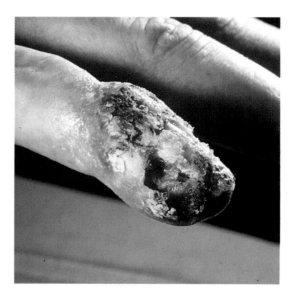

Subungual Malignant Melanoma

When a malignant melanoma is localized beneath the nail plate diagnosis may prove difficult. A subungual hematoma is capable of producing the same blue, red and white "tricolore" sign as that typically seen in malignant melanoma. A pigmented band may be a melanocytic nevus or a subungual fibroma but also the presenting sign of a malignant melanoma.

Malignant melanoma forms a tumour in the nail bed which is usually pigmented and gradually elevates and destroys the overlying nail plate. Pigment may spread to the surrounding skin, a phenomenon known as Hutchinson's sign.

Therapy consists in amputation of the finger or toe.

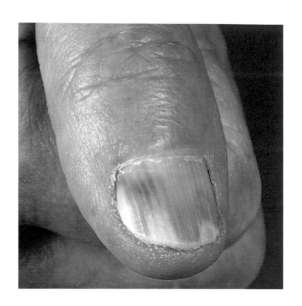

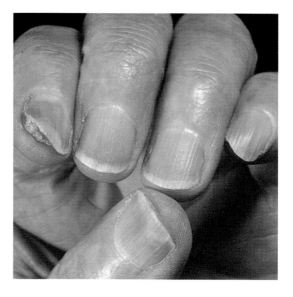

Subungual Lymphoma

Malignant, cutaneous lymphomas, B- as well as T-cell lymphomas may be seated subungually. Their initial presentation is a plaque in the nail bed resulting in onycholysis. Later a soft tumour is formed which destroys the nail plate.

Treatment consists of radiotherapy or chemotherapy.

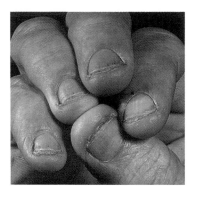

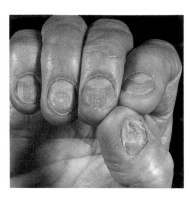

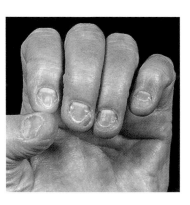

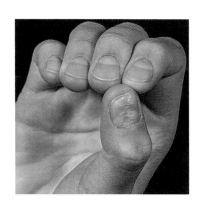

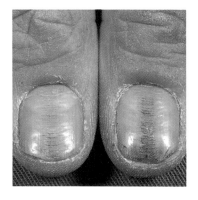

Onychotillomania

Habitual biting or manipulation of the finger nails and their surroundings is very common. It is by no means indicative of psychiatric disease but should rather be regarded as a bad habit. When the nail plate is bitten down, the exposed hyponychion forms a swelling at the fingertip. Manipulation of the proximal or lateral nail folds may also cause severe nail deformity (upper, middle left).

Median nail dystrophy, which is quite common, is usually located on one of the thumb nails and is caused by habitual, repeated manipulation of the middle part of the proximal nail fold. As a result, this nail fold is swollen and the cuticula are absent (middle right, bottom).

Index

D
Darier's disease 59
dermatomyositis 51, 53, 55, 57
drug eruptions 31

E
eczema 21
endocarditis lenta 21
erythroderma 45
exostoses 77, 79

F
fibroma 75, 81
fungal infections 15, 19

G
graft-versus-host reaction 9
griseofulvin 15

H
Hailey-Hailey's disease 59
half-and-half nails 25, 37, 67
hemorrhage 7, 21, 29, 67, 81
Hutchinson's sign 81
hyperhidrosis 19

I
ingrowing toe nails 39
iron deficiency 23, 49
itraconazole 15

pitting 7, 13
pityriasis rubra pilaris 11, 21
porphyria cutanea tarda 19
Pseudomonas 17, 29
psoriasis 7, 15, 19, 21, 43, 61, 65
pterygium 9
pterygium inversum 51, 53, 55, 57
pustular psoriasis 7
PUVA 7, 19
PUVA nails 29

R
radiotherapy 29
Raynaud's phenomenon 49, 51, 57
red lunulae 13, 31, 55
Reiter's disease 61
retinoid nails 69
retinoids 1, 7, 9, 59

S
scleroderma 9, 49, 57
splinters 7, 21
spoon nails 49, 57
squamous cell carcinoma 79
Staphylococcus aureus 15

T
terbinafine 15
Terry nails 25
thyreotoxicosis 19, 49
thyreotropic syndrome 47
trachyonychia 7, 43
Trichophyton rubrum 15
trumpet nails 45